YOUR KNOWLEDGE HAS VALUE

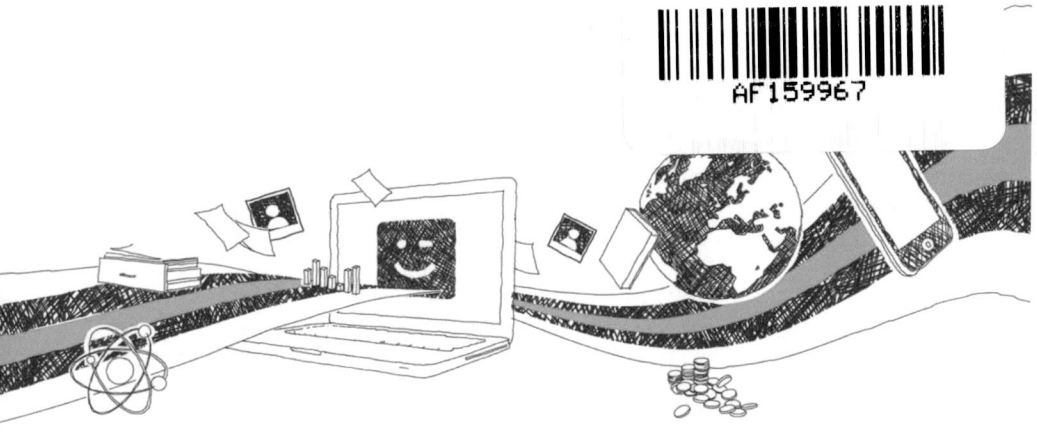

- We will publish your bachelor's and master's thesis, essays and papers

- Your own eBook and book - sold worldwide in all relevant shops

- Earn money with each sale

Upload your text at www.GRIN.com
and publish for free

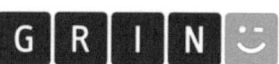

Bibliographic information published by the German National Library:

The German National Library lists this publication in the National Bibliography; detailed bibliographic data are available on the Internet at http://dnb.dnb.de .

This book is copyright material and must not be copied, reproduced, transferred, distributed, leased, licensed or publicly performed or used in any way except as specifically permitted in writing by the publishers, as allowed under the terms and conditions under which it was purchased or as strictly permitted by applicable copyright law. Any unauthorized distribution or use of this text may be a direct infringement of the author s and publisher s rights and those responsible may be liable in law accordingly.

Imprint:

Copyright © 2018 GRIN Verlag
Print and binding: Books on Demand GmbH, Norderstedt Germany
ISBN: 9783668628748

This book at GRIN:

https://www.grin.com/document/388557

Patrick Kimuyu

Sepsis Management. How to treat Sepsis in pharmacological and non-pharmacological ways

GRIN Verlag

GRIN - Your knowledge has value

Since its foundation in 1998, GRIN has specialized in publishing academic texts by students, college teachers and other academics as e-book and printed book. The website www.grin.com is an ideal platform for presenting term papers, final papers, scientific essays, dissertations and specialist books.

Visit us on the internet:

http://www.grin.com/

http://www.facebook.com/grincom

http://www.twitter.com/grin_com

Sepsis Management

Name: Patrick Kimuyu

INTRODUCTION

Sepsis is believed to be one of the most life-threatening medical conditions. This condition is associated with an infection that triggers inflammation responses leading to inflammations in different body parts and organs. In most cases, bacterial infections serve as the causes of sepsis. In practice, sepsis can be viewed as a condition that occur in three stages with sepsis progressing into severe sepsis and then septic shock that is characterized by organ failure. Evidence indicates that incidences for severe sepsis and septic shock have increased rapidly in the past decade and this is attributable to the increase of the aging population. As a result, severe sepsis and septic shock are considered some of the most causes of mortality and morbidity in intensive care (Claessens & Dhainaut, 2007). This phenomenon has prompted physicians and professional societies to implement management procedures that focus on early intervention. Therefore, this presentation will provide a comprehensive discussion on pharmacological and non pharmacological treatment of sepsis.

Objectives:
1. To create understanding on international sepsis management guidelines.
2. To create understanding on appropriate interventions in the management of sepsis.
3. To enable nurses to offer evidence-based practices and patient-centered care.

Prognosis of Sepsis

Prognosis of sepsis is based on systemic inflammatory response (SIRS) criteria. This implies that a patient should show at least two of the following signs and symptoms:

- Body temperature either low (<36^0 C or 96.8 F) or high (>38^0 C or 100.4 F)
- Elevated heart rate of more than 90 beats per minute
- Reduced $PaCO_2$ in arterial blood or respiratory rate of more than 20 breaths per minute
- White blood cell count of <4,000 cells/μL or >12,000 cells/μL

On the other hand, severity of sepsis is evaluated by the use of the MEDS (Mortality in Emergency Department Sepsis) score (Davis & Stöppler, 2015).

PHARMACOLOGICAL AND NON PHARMACOLOGICAL TREATMENT OF SEPSIS

Sepsis is associated with life-threatening outcomes, especially multiple organ failure. Therefore, the rationales for sepsis treatment are: eradication of infection, restoration of perfusion and maintenance of adequate organ function. Therefore, the following interventions ensure the goals and principles of sepsis treatment are met, primarily in treatment of severe sepsis and septic shock.

EARLY MANAGEMENT

Respiration Support

Patients with sepsis require respiratory support to prevent encephalopathy. Therefore, respiration can is stabilized through the use of supplemental oxygen. Intubation and mechanical ventilation are recommended for patients with dyspnea, persistent hypotension and inadequate peripheral perfusion (Kalil, 2015).

Assessment of Perfusion

Adequacy of perfusion is assessed after the stabilization of respiration. Inadequate perfusion is indicated by hypotension and elevated lactate. Systolic blood pressure of <90 mmHg and mean arterial pressure of <70 mmHg are characteristics of hypotension, whereas elevated serum lactate above 2 mmol/L reveal organ hypoperfusion.

Establishment of Venous Access

For patients with suspected sepsis, either peripheral or central venous access is required. Venous access is used for initial resuscitation and infusion of medication, fluids and blood products during the course of treatment (Schmidt & Mandel, 2015).

Urinary Catheterization

Urinary catheterization is meant to monitor renal function. In practice, urine output serves as a marker for adequate cardiac output and renal function. Normal urine output ranges from 30 to 50 mL/hr in adults. This is equivalent to 0.5 mL/kg/hr (Dellinger et al., 2013).

Fluid Resuscitation

The rationale for fluid resuscitation is to restore perfusion. Patients with sepsis experience intravascular hypovolemia; thus fluid resuscitation with intravenous fluids, primarily crystalloids is required. Other intravenous fluids that can be used are albumin solution, hydroxyethyl starch and pentastarch, although there is no conventional consensus that these colloid solutions have more benefits than crystalloid solutions (Schmidt & Mandel, 2015). In fluid resuscitation, patients should be monitored for signs of volume overload. These signs of volume overload include crackles on auscultation, dyspnea, pulmonary edema, and elevated jugular venous pressure (Kalil, 2015).

Early goal-directed therapy (EGDT): this therapy involves the administration of intravenous fluid following physiologic targets. It is done within the first 6 hours of sepsis presentation. EGDT seems to have gained an unprecedented acceptance in clinical practice. The main physiologic targets include MAP (mean arterial pressure) of ≥ 65 mmHg, CVP (central venous pressure) of 8 to 12 mmHg, urine output of ≥ 0.5 mL/kg/hr, and oxyhemoglobin saturation in central venous ($ScvO_2$) of more than 70% (Schmidt & Mandel, 2015).

Vasopressor Therapy

The rationale for the administration of vasopressors is to enhance blood flow distribution and reverse pathologic vasodilation through altering the activity of vascular smooth muscles. Vasopressor therapy is recommended for septic patients who do not respond to high volumes of isotonic crystalloid infusion.

During vasopressor therapy, norepinephrine and dopamine are administered as first-line agents, whereas epinephrine and phenylephrine are used as second-line agents.

In septic shock, antidiuretic hormone (ADH) or vasopressin is recommended owing to its depressed levels. It is also an endogenous peptide (Kalil, 2015).

Inotropic Therapy

Inotropic therapy is required for patients with severe and septic shock. The rationale for this therapy is to maintain cardiac output, especially in patients with refractory shock. Dobutamine, an inotropic agent increases cardiac output through rising blood pressure. It does so by decreasing peripheral vascular resistance.

Red Blood Cell Transfusions

Red blood cell transfusions are meant to increase hemoglobin level in critically-ill patients. In some cases, severe sepsis and septic shock are associated with active myocardial ischemia or hemorrhagic shock. Therefore, transfusion is recommended for patients with low hemoglobin level to raise it above 7 g/dL (Schmidt & Mandel, 2015).

CONTROL OF THE SEPTIC FOCUS

Identification of the Septic Focus (Diagnosis)

The rationale for this approach is to identify the etiology and site of infection for primary therapeutic interventions. Diagnostic tests reveal the infectious agent, problems in blood clotting, decreased oxygen saturation in blood, electrolyte imbalance, and organ function, primarily the liver and kidneys.

Results of blood tests may suggest further tests including urine test to identify urinary tract infection or mucus secretion test to identify the type of infectious agent causing the infection.

In cases where blood and culture tests do not show the infection, advanced diagnostic procedures can be performed including X-rays (check problem in lungs), CT scans (identify infections in internal organs such as pancreas, bowel area or appendix), ultrasound (identify infections in ovaries and gallbladder), and MRI to check infection in soft tissues (O'Connell, 2012).

Antimicrobial Therapy

Antimicrobial therapy aims at eradicating the infection. This therapy should be initiated within the first 6 hours after presentation following appropriate identification of the etiological agent. It is reported that mortality is reduced when antibiotic therapy is initiated early (Gaieski et al., 2010).

Beta-lactam agents such as cefotaxime, ampicillin or ceftriaxone in combination with a macrolide are administered to patients with community-acquired pneumonia.

ADDITIONAL THERAPIES

Corticosteroid Therapy

The rationale for corticosteroid therapy is to control inflammation. Ordinarily, sepsis involves intense inflammatory response. Therefore, corticosteroids such as glucocorticoid, hydrocortisone and fludrocortisone reduce treat inflammation. Hydrocortisone 100 mg IV is the most common choice (Kalil, 2015).

Intensive Insulin Therapy

The rationale for insulin therapy is glycemic control. This is so because patients with severe sepsis and septic shock experience insulin resistance and hyperglycemia. Therefore, glycemic control approaches should aim at maintaining glucose levels below 180 mg/dL (Kalil, 2015).

Surgical Treatment

Surgery is meant to drain soft tissue abscess and removal of sites of infection. In patients with septic shock, the common foci of infection are empyema, intra-abdominal sepsis, cholangitis, mediastinitis, pyelonephritis, septic arthritis, necrotizing fasciitis, and perirectal abscess (Kalil, 2015).

CONCLUSION

Sepsis is associated with high morbidity and mortality rates. It triggers whole-body inflammation that lead to multiple organ failure (Cassoobhoy, 2014). Therefore, interventions are aimed at eradicating infection, restoring perfusion and maintaining adequate organ function.

References

Cassoobhoy, A. (2014). *Sepsis (blood infection) and septic shock*. Retrieved from http://www.webmd.com/a-to-z-guides/sepsis-septicemia-blood-infection

Claessens, Y., & Dhainaut, J. (2007). Diagnosis and treatment of severe sepsis. *Crit Care*, 11(5): S2. doi: 10.1186/cc6153

Davis, C., & Stöppler, M. (2015). *Sepsis*. Retrieved from http://www.medicinenet.com/sepsis/article.htm

Dellinger, R., Levy, M., Rhodes, A., Annane, D., Gerlach, H., & Opal, S. (2013). Surviving sepsis campaign: international guidelines for management of severe sepsis and septic shock: 2012. *Crit Care Med.*, 41(2):580-637.

Gaieski, D., Mikkelsen, M., Band, R., Pines, J., Massone, R., Furia, F., Shofer, F., & Goyal, M. (2010). Impact of time to antibiotics on survival in patients with severe sepsis or septic shock in whom early goal-directed therapy was initiated in the emergency department. *Crit Care Med.*, 38:1045.

Kalil, A. (2015). *Septic shock treatment & management*. Retrieved from http://emedicine.medscape.com/article/168402-treatment#showall

O'Connell, K. (2012). *Sepsis*. Retrieved from http://www.healthline.com/health/sepsis#Overview1

Schmidt, G., & Mandel, J. (2015). *Evaluation and management of severe sepsis and septic shock in adults*. Retrieved from http://www.uptodate.com/contents/evaluation-and-management-of-severe-sepsis-and-septic-shock-in-adults

YOUR KNOWLEDGE HAS VALUE

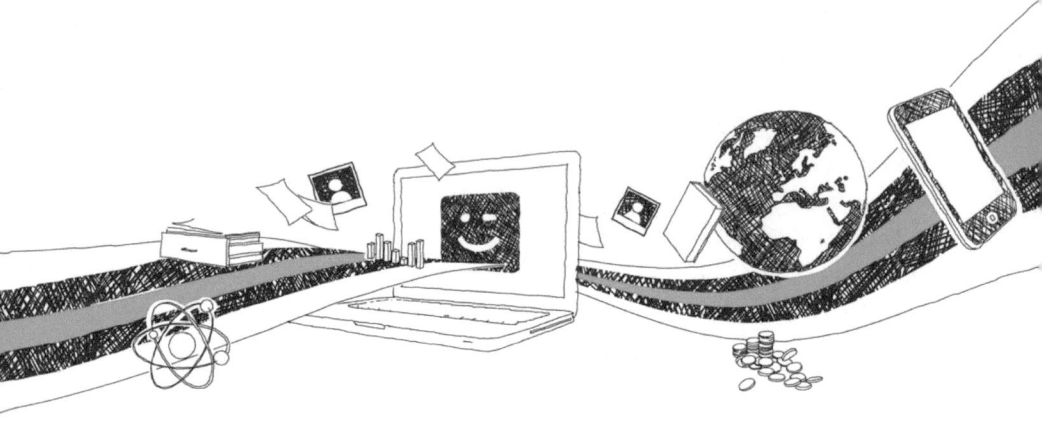

- We will publish your bachelor's and master's thesis, essays and papers

- Your own eBook and book - sold worldwide in all relevant shops

- Earn money with each sale

Upload your text at www.GRIN.com and publish for free

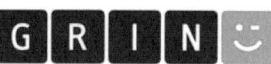